Pilates For Women Over 50

The Ultimate Beginners Guide for Women in Their Fifties and Beyond: Transforming Your Health to Rejuvenate Your Body and Mind

Juanita T. Williams

INTRODUCTION

In an era where age is increasingly celebrated for the wisdom and experience it brings, staying active and healthy has become a vital aspiration for many. This rings especially true for women over the age of 50, a stage of life where wellness and vitality take center stage.

Pilates, an exercise system designed to enhance flexibility, strength, and overall well-being, emerges as a beacon of hope for women in this demographic.

Welcome to "Pilates for Women Over 50," a comprehensive guide tailored to address the unique needs and concerns of mature women embarking on a journey towards better health and an enriched life through Pilates.

Welcome to Pilates for Women Over 50

As we step into the world of Pilates for women over 50, we extend a warm embrace, recognizing the distinctive path this age group traverses. It's a phase marked by wisdom, grace, and a deeper understanding of oneself.

Pilates offers a holistic approach to health, combining elements of strength, flexibility, balance, and mental well-being. This guide aims to seamlessly integrate Pilates into the lives of women over 50, considering their bodies, experiences, and aspirations.

Pilates is more than a physical exercise regimen; it's a philosophy that harmonizes the mind and body. Women over 50 often seek ways to maintain youthful vigor and stay active in a manner that respects their bodies' changing needs.

Pilates, with its low-impact yet highly effective exercises, provides precisely that.

It's about enhancing mobility, building muscle strength, improving posture, and promoting a sense of inner tranquility.

Understanding the Benefits of Pilates For You

The benefits of Pilates for women over 50 are diverse and impactful, encompassing physical, mental, and emotional aspects. The gentle yet challenging movements of Pilates help counteract the effects of aging, fostering a stronger and more resilient body.

Muscles that might have weakened over the years can be revitalized, contributing to better posture and reduced discomfort.

Pilates also places a strong emphasis on core strength and stability. This is particularly beneficial for women in this age group as it supports the spine and can alleviate issues related to back pain or discomfort.

Additionally, the focus on breath control and mindfulness in Pilates helps in managing stress and promoting mental clarity, essential components of overall well-being, especially for women experiencing the various facets of life post-50.

Moreover, Pilates is adaptable to various fitness levels and health conditions. Whether you're new to exercise or a seasoned fitness enthusiast, Pilates can be tailored to suit your abilities and requirements.

For women over 50, this adaptability is key, allowing them to engage in exercises that align with their physical condition and goals.

What to Expect from this Book

In "Pilates for Women Over 50," we have meticulously structured the content to serve as a comprehensive roadmap for your journey through Pilates. Expect to embark on a transformative experience that not only nurtures your body but also cultivates a positive mindset.

The book encompasses a holistic approach, covering the foundational principles of Pilates, key exercises, modifications for varying fitness levels, tips for safety and injury prevention, and insights into nutrition that complements your Pilates practice.

Each chapter has been crafted with you in mind, considering your unique needs, concerns, and goals. Whether you're looking to improve flexibility, enhance strength, alleviate discomfort, or simply revitalize your spirit, our aim is to guide you through a tailored Pilates experience.

Together, let's embrace this enriching journey through the realms of Pilates, tailored for the vibrant and dynamic women over 50. Let us build strength, grace, and vitality hand in hand, celebrating the beauty of this unique life stage.

Here's to discovering the transformative power of Pilates and embracing the best version of yourself.

PILATES AND AGING: A PERFECT MATCH

Pilates emerges as a perfect match for the aging population due to its low-impact nature, focus on core strength, flexibility enhancement, and mental well-being.

How Aging Affects the Body

The aging process impacts the human body in various ways, presenting both visible and invisible changes. Starting at the cellular level, aging brings about a decrease in the production of important substances such as collagen and elastin, resulting in reduced skin elasticity and firmness.

Bones and muscles tend to weaken and lose density, which can lead to increased frailty and a higher risk of fractures. Joints may experience a reduction in lubrication and flexibility, making movement more challenging. Additionally, the metabolism slows down, making weight management increasingly difficult.

As aging affects the body, it can also impact mental and emotional health. Cognitive decline and the risk of neurodegenerative diseases rise with age, potentially leading to issues with memory, cognitive function, and mental clarity.

Emotional well-being can also be affected, with factors like retirement, empty nesting, or loss of loved ones contributing to feelings of isolation or sadness.

Why Pilates is Ideal for You

Here's why Pilates is particularly well-suited for women in this age group:

Low Impact:
Pilates exercises are gentle on the joints and muscles, making them perfect for those dealing with joint pain, arthritis, or other mobility issues that often accompany aging.

The controlled movements ensure a reduced risk of injury.

Improved Flexibility:
Aging often leads to a decrease in flexibility, affecting mobility and overall comfort. Pilates focuses on elongating and stretching muscles, thus enhancing flexibility and range of motion.

Muscle Strength and Tone:
Loss of muscle mass is a common concern with aging. Pilates, emphasizing resistance and bodyweight exercises, helps in building and toning muscles, promoting strength and stability.

Enhanced Posture:
As people age, maintaining good posture becomes essential to prevent back problems and maintain spinal health. Pilates exercises concentrate on improving posture through awareness and strengthening of the core muscles.

Focus on Balance:
Balance tends to decline with age, making individuals more susceptible to falls. Pilates incorporates exercises that improve balance and coordination, reducing the risk of falls and related injuries.

Mental Well-being:
Pilates promotes mindfulness and concentration through deliberate, flowing movements. This aids in reducing stress, improving mental clarity, and enhancing overall well-being, crucial aspects for older adults.

Adaptability:
Pilates exercises can be modified to suit varying fitness levels and health conditions, making it inclusive and accessible to women over 50, regardless of their current physical state.

Common Concerns and How Pilates Addresses Them

Osteoporosis and Bone Health:
Women over 50 are often concerned about bone density and osteoporosis. Pilates, incorporating weight-bearing exercises, aids in building bone density, reducing the risk of fractures and enhancing overall bone health.

Joint Pain and Arthritis:
Joint pain and arthritis are prevalent concerns with aging. Pilates, being low-impact and adaptable, helps alleviate joint pain by providing gentle movements that promote joint flexibility and strength.

Weight Management:
Metabolism slows down with age, making weight management challenging. Pilates, by promoting lean muscle mass and aiding in burning calories, supports weight management efforts in a sustainable manner.

Back Pain:
Back pain often becomes more prevalent as individuals age. Pilates focuses on strengthening the core and back muscles, enhancing posture, and reducing the occurrence and intensity of back pain.

GETTING STARTED WITH PILATES

This section will guide you through the essential steps to commence your Pilates practice, ensuring a safe, enjoyable, and fulfilling experience.

Assessing Your Fitness Level

Before diving into Pilates, it's essential to assess your current fitness level. Understanding where you stand regarding strength, flexibility, balance, and overall fitness will help tailor your Pilates routine to meet your specific needs and capabilities.

Strength Assessment:
- Evaluate your muscular strength by gauging how many repetitions of bodyweight exercises (e.g., push-ups, squats) you can comfortably perform.

- Assess specific muscle groups, including core, upper body, lower body, and back muscles.

Flexibility and Range of Motion:
- Measure your flexibility by attempting basic stretches, like touching your toes or reaching overhead.
- Observe your range of motion in major joints such as hips, shoulders, and spine.

Balance and Coordination:
- Stand on one leg to assess your balance and stability. Note how long you can maintain your balance and how steady you feel.

Cardiovascular Fitness:
- Consider your endurance and cardiovascular fitness, though Pilates is not primarily a cardiovascular workout.

Any Physical Limitations:
- Acknowledge any pre-existing injuries, medical conditions, or physical limitations that may affect your ability to perform certain exercises.

Consulting a Healthcare Professional

Before initiating any exercise program, including Pilates, it is prudent to seek advice from a healthcare professional, especially if you have underlying health concerns or medical conditions.

Consult with your primary care physician or a relevant specialist to ensure that Pilates is suitable for your current health status.

Medical History Discussion:
- Share your medical history, including past injuries, surgeries, chronic

conditions, or medications, with your healthcare provider.

Exercise Recommendations:

- Request recommendations or restrictions on exercise activities, considering your health condition.

Exercise Safety Guidelines:

- Receive guidance on exercising safely, addressing any concerns or precautions related to Pilates.

Exercise Modifications:

- Seek advice on specific exercises that may need to be modified or avoided based on your health status.

Setting Realistic Goals

- Establishing clear and achievable goals is a pivotal step towards a successful Pilates journey. Setting realistic objectives will help keep you motivated and focused throughout your practice.

Short-term Goals:
- Set attainable goals for the upcoming weeks or months, such as increasing your workout frequency or mastering a particular Pilates exercise.

Long-term Goals:
- Envision your fitness aspirations in the long run, be it enhancing overall flexibility, improving core strength, or achieving a specific level of mastery in Pilates.

Measurable Goals:
- Ensure your goals are quantifiable and measurable so that progress can be tracked and celebrated.

Realistic and Achievable Goals:
- Align your goals with your fitness level and lifestyle, ensuring they are achievable within a reasonable timeframe.

Revising Goals:
- Be open to modifying your goals as you progress, adapting them to your evolving fitness level and newfound Pilates abilities.

UNDERSTANDING THE PRINCIPLES OF PILATES

Understanding and embodying these principles are essential to gaining maximum benefit from your Pilates practice. They contribute not only to physical progress but also to mental clarity, mindfulness, and a deeper connection with your body.

The Six Principles of Pilates: A Detailed Overview

Joseph Pilates, the creator of the Pilates method, established six fundamental principles that are woven into every exercise and aspect of Pilates.

These principles are the cornerstone of the practice, emphasizing the integration of mind and body to achieve a harmonious and efficient movement.

Breathing:

- **Description**: Proper breathing is considered the cornerstone of the Pilates method. It's a vital aspect that aids in enhancing oxygen circulation, improving lung capacity, and promoting relaxation during exercises.

- **Technique**: Pilates breathing involves lateral thoracic breathing, engaging the diaphragm to inhale deeply through the nose and exhale fully through the mouth.

Concentration:

- **Description**: Concentration is about focusing your mind entirely on the exercise you're performing. It's a deliberate mental effort to connect with each movement, muscle, and breath.

- **Technique**: Direct your attention to the specific muscles being used, the alignment of your body, and the precision of each movement. A focused mind facilitates a purposeful and effective workout.

Control:

- **Description**: Control is about executing movements with precision and awareness. It involves maintaining a smooth and deliberate pace, ensuring every part of the body is engaged and controlled throughout the exercise.

- **Technique**: Avoid rushed or erratic movements. Perform each exercise with a sense of control, activating the relevant muscles and maintaining proper alignment.

Centering:

- **Description**: Centering is the concept of drawing your focus and energy to the body's center, often referred to as the powerhouse or core. This area is essential for initiating and sustaining movements effectively.

- **Technique**: Engage your deep abdominal muscles, pelvic floor, and lower back muscles to establish a strong center. Movements in Pilates typically start from this powerhouse.

Precision:

- **Description**: Precision emphasizes the accuracy and exactness in performing each movement. It involves executing exercises with the correct alignment, muscle engagement, and intended range of motion.

- **Technique**: Pay careful attention to the details of every movement, ensuring proper form and muscle activation. Even slight adjustments can significantly impact the effectiveness of the exercise.

Flow:

- **Description**: Flow refers to the seamless and continuous movement through a series of exercises. It encourages grace, fluidity, and connectivity between different movements.

- **Technique**: Aim for a smooth transition from one exercise to another, maintaining a consistent pace and rhythm. Flow allows for a dynamic and uninterrupted Pilates session.

Now, let's explore each of these principles in more detail, emphasizing their significance and how they can be applied effectively during your Pilates practice.

Breathing

Breathing is a fundamental principle in Pilates that plays a crucial role in enhancing the quality and effectiveness of the exercises. Proper breathing not only oxygenates the body but also promotes relaxation, concentration, and muscle engagement.

Role of Breathing:

- **Oxygenation**: Deep, diaphragmatic breathing facilitates efficient oxygen intake, providing the muscles with the necessary oxygen for optimal performance.

- **Relaxation**: Controlled breathing aids in relaxation, reducing tension in muscles and promoting a calm mental state during exercises.

- **Core Engagement**: The act of breathing deeply engages the core muscles, especially the transverse abdominis and pelvic floor muscles, supporting stability and control.

Breathing Technique:

- **Lateral Thoracic Breathing**: Inhale deeply through the nose, allowing the ribs to expand laterally and the chest to rise. Exhale fully through the mouth, allowing the ribs to contract and the chest to lower.

- **Ribcage Expansion**: As you inhale, visualize expanding the rib cage in all directions front, back, sides promoting a three-dimensional breath.

Incorporating Breath into Pilates:

- **Coordinate with Movements**: Sync your breath with the movement. Inhale during the preparatory phase or the easier part of the exercise and exhale during the exertion or challenging phase.

- **Maintain a Rhythmic Pattern**: Establish a consistent and rhythmic breathing pattern throughout your Pilates routine, ensuring a steady flow of oxygen to the muscles.

- **Focused Breath Observation**: Direct your attention to your breath, noticing its depth, rhythm, and how it moves within your body during exercises.

- **Calming Effect**: Paying attention to your breath can be a meditative practice, calming the mind and promoting mental clarity during your Pilates session.

Concentration

Concentration in Pilates embodies the principle of mind-body connection, emphasizing the need to be fully present and engaged during each movement. It encourages a focused and deliberate approach to exercise, enhancing precision and effectiveness.

Role of Concentration:

- **Enhanced Awareness**: Concentration directs your

awareness to the muscles being engaged, the alignment of your body, and the specific movement you are performing.

- **Mind-Body Unity:** By concentrating on the task at hand, you create a strong connection between your mind and body, fostering a deeper understanding of your movements and their effects.

Techniques to Enhance Concentration:

- **Focus on Muscle Engagement**: Direct your attention to the muscle groups involved in the exercise, feeling their activation and engagement throughout the movement.

- **Visualize Movement**: Visualize the correct form and movement before executing it, enhancing mental preparation and aiding in precise execution.

- **Minimize Distractions**: Eliminate distractions and external noise during your Pilates practice to maintain a high level of concentration.

Incorporating Concentration into Pilates:

- **Mindful Movement**: Perform each exercise with complete awareness, ensuring that your mind is present and focused on the current movement and its execution.

- **Intentional Engagement**: Be intentional in engaging the correct muscles, initiating movement with purpose, and maintaining control throughout.

Benefits of Concentration:

- **Improved Performance**: Concentration enhances the effectiveness of each movement, allowing you to perform exercises more accurately and with better results.

- **Enhanced Mindfulness**: The mindful approach fosters mental clarity, reduces stress, and promotes a meditative state during your Pilates session.

Control

Control is a fundamental principle in Pilates that emphasizes deliberate and precise movements. It involves executing each exercise with mastery, focus, and the utmost control over every part of the body.

Role of Control:

- **Muscle Engagement**: Control ensures that the intended muscles are engaged throughout the movement, promoting muscle strength and endurance.

- **Stability and Balance**: Controlled movements aid in maintaining stability and balance, preventing any sudden or jerky actions that could lead to injuries.

Techniques to Enhance Control:

- Mindful Approach: Approach each exercise with a mindful mindset, focusing on each component of the movement and ensuring it is executed smoothly and with control.

- **Body Awareness**: Cultivate awareness of your body's alignment, muscle engagement, and movement, maintaining a sense of control over every part.

Incorporating Control into Pilates:

- **Gradual Progression**: Begin with simpler movements, mastering control over the basics, and gradually progress to more complex exercises, maintaining the same level of control.

Benefits of Control:

- **Injury Prevention**: Control minimizes the risk of injuries by ensuring that movements are deliberate, controlled, and within the body's safe range of motion.

- **Enhanced Muscle Tone**: Precise control over movements results in better muscle engagement, promoting muscle tone and strength.

Centering

Centering is a foundational principle in Pilates, emphasizing the importance of the body's center, often referred to as the powerhouse. The powerhouse comprises the core muscles and serves as the focal point for initiating movements and maintaining stability.

Role of Centering:

- **Initiating Movements**: The powerhouse is the primary area from where movements are initiated, providing strength and support for the entire body.

- **Stability and Balance**: A strong and engaged center stabilizes the body, improving balance and control during exercises.

Techniques to Engage the Center:

- **Abdominal Engagement**: Activate the deep abdominal muscles, particularly the transverse abdominis, by drawing the navel towards the spine.

- **Pelvic Floor Engagement**: Engage the pelvic floor muscles, lifting them slightly, to complete the powerhouse engagement.

Incorporating Centering into Pilates:

- **Initiate Movements from the Center**: Begin each exercise by engaging your powerhouse, ensuring that all movements originate from this central point.

- **Maintain Core Engagement**: Throughout the exercise, keep your center engaged to promote stability and control.

Benefits of Centering:

- **Enhanced Core Strength**: Centering promotes a strong core by encouraging consistent engagement of the abdominal and pelvic floor muscles.

- **Improved Posture**: Engaging the center aids in maintaining proper posture during exercises and daily activities.

Precision

Precision is a fundamental principle in Pilates that emphasizes executing movements with exactness and accuracy. It involves attention to detail and a meticulous approach to each exercise, promoting optimal alignment and muscle engagement.

Role of Precision:

- **Muscle Isolation**: Precision encourages isolating specific muscles and engaging them precisely, preventing unnecessary muscle engagement and ensuring targeted work.

- **Proper Alignment**: Precise movements promote correct alignment of the body, reducing the risk of injuries and enhancing the effectiveness of the exercise.

Techniques to Enhance Precision:

- **Mindful Awareness**: Focus on the form, alignment, and engagement of each muscle involved in the exercise, ensuring precise execution.

- **Visual Alignment Checks**: Use mirrors or visual cues to monitor your alignment and form during exercises, making necessary adjustments for accuracy.

Incorporating Precision into Pilates:

- **Attention to Detail**: Be meticulous in your approach, paying close attention to every movement, muscle engagement, and alignment, aiming for perfection in execution.

Benefits of Precision:

- **Maximized Effectiveness**: Precise movements target specific muscle groups effectively, promoting muscle strength, tone, and flexibility.

- **Reduced Risk of Injury**: By focusing on accurate alignment and form, precision minimizes the risk of strain or injury during exercises.

Flow

Flow, a core principle in Pilates, emphasizes the seamless and continuous transition between exercises and movements. It encourages a rhythmic and graceful flow, promoting a sense of harmony and connection throughout the practice.

Role of Flow:

- **Smooth Transitions**: Flow facilitates smooth transitions between exercises, creating a sense of continuity and rhythm in your Pilates routine.

- **Increased Flexibility:** A flowing practice encourages fluidity in movements, enhancing flexibility and agility.

Techniques to Enhance Flow:

- **Maintain a Steady Pace**: Maintain a consistent and even pace throughout your Pilates session, ensuring a continuous flow of movements.

- **Connect Movements**: Seamlessly connect one exercise to the next, avoiding abrupt stops or jerky transitions.

Incorporating Flow into Pilates:

- **Focus on Rhythm**: Sync your movements to a rhythmic pattern, creating a natural flow that carries you from one exercise to another.

Benefits of Flow:

- **Enhanced Mind-Body Connection**: Flow promotes a heightened sense of connection between your mind and body, fostering a meditative state during your Pilates practice.

- **Elevated Exercise Experience**: A flowing practice elevates the overall experience, making your Pilates routine more enjoyable and satisfying.

EQUIPMENT AND ACCESSORIES

Essential Pilates Equipment For You

The Reformer:

Description: The Reformer is perhaps the most versatile and iconic piece of Pilates equipment. It consists of a carriage that slides on rails, springs for resistance, and various straps and bars to facilitate a wide range of exercises.

Benefits For You:
- **Low Impact**: The Reformer provides a low-impact workout, reducing stress on joints, making it suitable for women experiencing age-related joint concerns.

- **Muscle Tone**: It offers comprehensive muscle toning,

particularly targeting the core, which is vital for maintaining posture and supporting the spine.

- **Flexibility**: The Reformer supports flexibility training, aiding in maintaining or improving range of motion, crucial for maintaining an active lifestyle as you age.

Stability Balls:

Description: Stability balls, also known as Swiss balls or exercise balls, are large, inflatable balls used for a variety of Pilates exercises to challenge stability, balance, and muscle engagement.

Benefits For You:
- **Core Strengthening**: Stability balls engage the core muscles effectively, aiding in strengthening the abdominal and lower back muscles, vital for posture and spinal support.

- **Balance and Stability**: They improve balance and stability, reducing the risk of falls and enhancing confidence in movement, which is particularly important for older adults.

- **Versatility**: Stability balls add versatility to exercises, allowing for modifications and variations that cater to different fitness levels and needs.

Resistance Bands:

Description: Resistance bands are elastic bands available in varying strengths, providing resistance to your movements during Pilates exercises.

Benefits For You:
- **Gentle Strength Training**: Resistance bands offer a gentle yet effective way to engage muscles and build strength without putting excessive stress on joints.

- **Improved Muscle Tone**: They contribute to improved muscle tone, enhancing overall body strength and helping combat muscle loss associated with aging.

- **Portability**: Resistance bands are portable and versatile, making them convenient for home workouts or when traveling.

Magic Circle:

Description: The magic circle, also known as a Pilates ring or exercise ring, is a circular ring made of flexible metal or rubber with padded handles. It is used for various resistance exercises in Pilates.

Benefits For You:
- Targeted Muscle Engagement: The magic circle provides targeted resistance, aiding in engaging specific muscle groups, including the inner thighs, arms, and chest.

- **Enhanced Flexibility**: Incorporating the magic circle into exercises can help improve flexibility, particularly in areas like the hips and shoulders, which tend to stiffen with age.

- **Added Challenge**: It adds a challenge to exercises, making workouts more engaging and promoting increased muscle engagement.

Choosing the Right Equipment for Your Needs

When selecting Pilates equipment for your workouts, particularly as a woman over 50, it's crucial to consider your fitness goals, preferences, any existing health conditions, and your overall Pilates experience level. Here are key factors to guide you in choosing the right equipment:

Fitness Goals:

- **Strength and Toning**: If your primary goal is to build strength and tone muscles, equipment like the

Reformer and resistance bands would be excellent choices.

- **Flexibility**: For improving flexibility and range of motion, stability balls and the magic circle can be highly effective.

- **Overall Fitness**: If you're looking for a versatile piece of equipment for a well-rounded workout, consider a Reformer, which offers a wide range of exercises.

Health and Safety:
- **Low Impact**: If you have joint concerns or are looking for low-impact exercises, the Reformer and stability balls are gentle on the joints while providing an effective workout.

- **Mobility**: Consider your mobility level and choose equipment that complements your mobility while still challenging you appropriately.

Space and Storage:

- **Home Space**: If you have limited space at home, opt for equipment that is compact, foldable, or easy to store, like resistance bands and stability balls.

- **Portability**: If you travel frequently or want to exercise on the go, choose portable equipment such as resistance bands or a collapsible Reformer.

Budget:

- **Cost-effective Options**: If you have budget constraints, stability balls and resistance bands are cost-effective yet versatile choices that provide a range of exercises.

Comfort and Preference:

- **Personal Comfort**: Consider your comfort level and preference for specific equipment. Some individuals may find certain equipment more comfortable and enjoyable to use.

Consult a Professional:

- **Trainer's Advice:** Seek advice from a certified Pilates trainer or healthcare professional to ensure you choose equipment that aligns with your needs and abilities.

KEY PILATES EXERCISES FOR YOU

Warm-Up and Cool-Down Stretches

Warm-Up Stretches: Neck Stretch:

Description: Gently tilt your head to the side, bringing your ear towards your shoulder, holding the stretch to release neck tension.

Benefits:
- Relieves neck stiffness, common in individuals with sedentary jobs.

- Enhances neck mobility and flexibility.

Shoulder Rolls:

Description: Roll your shoulders forward and backward in a circular motion, loosening up the shoulder muscles.

Benefits:
- Reduces shoulder tension and stiffness.

- Improves circulation and warms up the upper body.

Cat-Cow Stretch:

Description: Transition between arching your back upward (cat) and dipping your back downward (cow), coordinating with your breath.

Benefits:
- Mobilizes the spine and stretches the back muscles.

- Enhances flexibility and alignment.

Cool-Down Stretches: Spinal Twist:

Description: Sit or lie down and gently twist your torso to one side, holding the stretch for a few breaths before switching sides.

Benefits:

- Relieves tension in the back and spine.

- Improves spinal mobility and flexibility.

Hamstring Stretch:

Description: Extend one leg and gently lean forward, reaching for your toes while keeping the leg straight.

Benefits:

- Stretches the hamstrings, essential for maintaining leg flexibility.

- Promotes better posture and reduces the risk of lower back issues.

Description: Sit back on your heels, extending your arms forward and lowering your chest towards the floor, reaching a resting pose.

Benefits:
- Relaxes the back, shoulders, and neck.

- Soothes the mind and supports stress alleviation.

Mat Exercises

The Hundred:

Description: Lie on your back, lift your head and legs, and pump your arms while inhaling for five counts and exhaling for five counts.

Benefits:
- Engages the core muscles and enhances cardiovascular endurance.

- Wakes up the body and improves circulation.

The Roll-Up:

Description: Start lying down, arms extended overhead. Roll up to a seated position, reaching towards your toes, then roll back down.

Benefits:
- Strengthens the core muscles, particularly the abdominals.

- Enhances spinal flexibility and control.

Single-Leg Circles:

Description: Lie on your back, lift one leg, and draw circles in the air with your toes.

Benefits:
- Works on pelvic stability and hip mobility.

- Tones and strengthens the lower abdominals and hip flexors.

Rolling Like a Ball:

Description: Balance on your sit bones, hug your knees, and roll back and forth, maintaining a rounded spine.

Benefits:
- Massages the spine and massages the back muscles.

- Challenges core stability and coordination.

The Saw:

Description: Seated with legs extended, twist your torso to reach one hand towards the opposite foot, then return to center and switch sides.

Benefits:
- Enhances spinal rotation and stretches the waist muscles.

- Works on abdominal strength and flexibility.

The Swan:

Description: Lie on your stomach, place your hands near your shoulders, and lift your upper body, arching your back.

Benefits:
- Strengthens the back muscles and improves posture.

- Stretches the chest and shoulders.

Leg Pulls:

Description: Start in a plank position and alternate lifting your legs, engaging your core and glutes.

Benefits:
- Enhances core strength, particularly targeting the abdominals.

- Improves overall body control and stability.

Reformer Exercises

Footwork Series:

Heel Raises:

Description: Press the balls of your feet on the foot bar and lift your heels, then lower them back down.

Benefits:
- Strengthens calf muscles and ankles.

- Aids in improving balance and foot alignment.

Arch Raises:

Description: Press the heels, keeping the balls of the feet on the bar, and lift the arches of the feet, then lower them back down.

Benefits:
- Strengthens the muscles along the arch of the foot.

- Assists in maintaining proper foot mechanics.

Knee Stretches:

Knee Flexion:

Description: Start in a plank position and bring your knees towards your chest, then extend them back out.

Benefits:
- Works the abdominals and enhances core stability.

- Improves hip flexor flexibility.

Pelvic Lift:

Bridge:

Description: Lie on your back, bend your knees, and lift your pelvis off the carriage, engaging your glutes and hamstrings.

Benefits:
- Strengthens the glutes, hamstrings, and lower back.

- Enhances spinal mobility and stability.

Mermaid:

Side Stretch:

Description: Sit sideways on the Reformer, extending one arm up and stretching to the side.

Benefits:
- Stretches the side body and engages the oblique muscles.

- Improves lateral flexibility and mobility.

Short Box Series:

Round Back:

Description: Sit on the box, round your spine, and articulate it down while engaging your abdominals.

Benefits:
- Strengthens the abdominal muscles and improves posture.

- Enhances spinal mobility and control.

Rowing Series:

Front Rowing:

Description: Sit on the Reformer, round your spine, and pull the straps towards your chest, then extend them forward.

Benefits:
- Works the upper back, shoulders, and arms.

- Promotes spinal flexibility and scapular stability.

DESIGNING YOUR PILATES ROUTINE

Here's a step-by-step guide to crafting your Pilates routine:

Determine Your Goals:
- **Ask yourself**: What do you want to achieve through Pilates? Is it improving flexibility, strengthening your core, rehabilitating an injury, or simply staying active and healthy?

- **Tailor exercises**: Based on your goals, select exercises that align with what you want to accomplish.

Assess Your Fitness Level:
- **Evaluate strengths and weaknesses**: Identify your fitness strengths and areas that need improvement, ensuring a balanced approach to your routine.

- **Consider modifications**: Choose exercises that match your fitness level, allowing for progression as you improve.

Select the Right Exercises:
- **Include variety**: Incorporate a mix of exercises targeting different muscle groups to ensure a comprehensive workout.

- **Progressive challenge:** Include exercises that challenge you progressively to promote growth and improvement.

Consider Equipment and Props:
- **Choose based on availability**: If you have access to Pilates equipment like a Reformer or stability ball, incorporate exercises that utilize them for added variety and challenge.

- **Adapt without equipment**: If equipment is limited, opt for mat exercises or those using resistance bands for an effective workout.

Plan the Routine:
- **Warm-up:** Begin with gentle warm-up stretches to prepare your body for the workout.

- **Exercise sequence**: Organize exercises logically, considering muscle groups and transitioning smoothly between movements.

- **Cool down**: Conclude with stretches to enhance flexibility and reduce muscle tension.

Focus on Form and Technique:
- **Prioritize proper form**: Emphasize maintaining correct form during exercises to ensure effectiveness and prevent injuries.

- **Mindful movement**: Practice mindful movement, paying attention to muscle engagement and breathing throughout each exercise.

Monitor and Adjust:

- **Regular assessments**: Assess your progress periodically and make necessary adjustments to the routine based on your achievements and goals.

- **Listen to your body**: Modify exercises or intensity based on how your body feels to prevent overexertion or injury.

Remember, your Pilates routine should be enjoyable and suited to your lifestyle. Feel free to experiment with different exercises and variations to find what works best for you.

Creating a Weekly Workout Schedule

Here's a comprehensive guide on how to create an effective weekly workout schedule:

Assess Your Time Commitment:
- **Determine available time:** Consider your daily and weekly schedule to identify time slots available for workouts.

- **Realistic commitment:** Be realistic about how much time you can dedicate to exercise each day.

Set Clear Fitness Goals:
- **Define your objectives:** Establish clear short-term and long-term fitness goals, whether it's weight loss, muscle gain, increased flexibility, or overall wellness.

- **Align with your schedule**: Ensure your goals align with the time you have available for workouts.

Plan a Balanced Workout Routine:
- **Incorporate variety**: Include a mix of cardio, strength training, flexibility, and recovery exercises throughout the week.

- **Prioritize recovery:** Allocate time for rest and recovery to prevent burnout and promote muscle healing.

Divide Your Weekly Schedule:
- **Daily focus:** Designate specific days for different types of workouts, such as cardio on Mondays, Pilates on Wednesdays, and yoga on Fridays.

- **Rotate muscle groups**: Alternate strength training days to allow specific muscle groups to recover and rebuild.

Gradually Increase Intensity:
- **Progressive overload**: Gradually increase the intensity, duration, or complexity of exercises as you progress, challenging your body and avoiding plateaus.

- **Periodization**: Implement periodization by organizing your workouts into cycles of varying intensities and volumes.

Consider Lifestyle Factors:
- **Work demands**: Adjust your workout schedule based on your work schedule, ensuring you have ample time for exercise without compromising work commitments.

- **Family and social obligations**: Coordinate your workouts around family activities and social events to maintain a balanced lifestyle.

Be Flexible and Adapt:
- **Expect the unexpected**: Be prepared to adapt your schedule

when unexpected events or commitments arise, and find alternative times for your workouts.

Track Your Progress:
- **Record achievements**: Keep a fitness journal to track your progress, noting improvements in strength, endurance, flexibility, or weight loss.

- **Celebrate milestones**: Celebrate your achievements and milestones to stay motivated and committed to your workout routine.

Incorporating Cardio and Aerobic Exercise

Cardiovascular or aerobic exercises are essential components of a well-rounded fitness routine. They enhance heart health, improve endurance, support weight management, and boost overall energy levels.

Integrating cardio into your Pilates routine offers a comprehensive workout that combines the benefits of both. Here's how to effectively incorporate cardio and aerobic exercises into your Pilates routine:

Understand Cardio Benefits:
- **Improved heart health**: Cardio exercises strengthen the heart muscle and improve blood circulation, reducing the risk of heart disease.

- **Calorie burning**: Aerobic activities help burn calories, aiding in weight management and fat loss.

- **Enhanced endurance**: Regular cardio improves endurance, allowing you to sustain longer and more intense workouts.

Choose Cardio Exercises:
- **Select activities you enjoy**: Opt for cardio exercises that you find enjoyable, whether it's running, cycling, dancing, swimming, or brisk walking.

- **Variety is key:** Incorporate a mix of high-intensity interval training (HIIT), moderate-intensity exercises, and low-impact options to keep your routine engaging.

Integrate Cardio into Your Pilates Routine:
- **Pre-Pilates cardio warm-up:** Begin your Pilates session with a short cardio warm-up, like jumping jacks or high knees, to increase heart rate and warm up muscles.

- **Interval training:** Combine intervals of cardio exercises with Pilates movements to elevate your heart rate, intensify the workout, and burn more calories.

Schedule Cardio Sessions:
- **Balanced approach:** Aim for at least 150 minutes of moderate-intensity aerobic activity or 75 minutes of vigorous-intensity

aerobic activity per week, spread across the week.

- **Mix with Pilates**: Incorporate cardio workouts 2-4 times a week, alongside Pilates sessions, to maintain balance and achieve your fitness goals.

Monitor Progress and Adjust:
- **Progressive intensity**: Gradually increase the intensity and duration of your cardio workouts to challenge your fitness level and continually improve.

- **Listen to your body**: Pay attention to how your body responds to cardio exercises and adapt accordingly, avoiding overexertion or injury.

Prioritize Recovery:
- **Post-cardio stretches**: After cardio sessions, incorporate gentle stretches to ease muscle tension and enhance flexibility, complementing the benefits of Pilates.

Stay Consistent and Enjoy the Process:
- **Consistent effort:** Stick to your cardio routine, ensuring you meet your weekly goals, and adjust your schedule as needed to accommodate other workouts.

- **Enjoy variety:** Explore different cardio activities to keep your workouts exciting and maintain motivation.

Adapting Pilates to Your Lifestyle

Here are key strategies to adapt Pilates to your lifestyle effectively:

Assess Your Lifestyle:
- **Analyze daily activities:** Evaluate your daily routine, considering work commitments, family responsibilities, and other obligations that shape your schedule.

- Identify time pockets: Pinpoint time slots that can be dedicated to Pilates without disrupting your existing commitments.

Incorporate Pilates Throughout the Day:
- **Micro-workouts**: Break your Pilates routine into shorter, manageable sessions throughout the day, such as 10-minute mini-Pilates workouts during breaks.

- **Integrate into daily tasks**: Practice Pilates principles, like engaging your core or focusing on posture, during everyday activities like walking, standing, or sitting at your desk.

Make Use of Technology:
- **Online Pilates classes**: Utilize online platforms or Pilates apps that offer a variety of classes, making it convenient to choose workouts that align with your schedule.

- **Set reminders**: Use alarms or reminders on your phone to prompt your Pilates sessions, ensuring you stay on track with your routine.

Customize Your Pilates Routine:
- **Tailored exercises:** Adapt your Pilates routine based on your preferences, fitness level, and any specific areas you want to target.

- **Incorporate favorite activities**: Combine Pilates with activities you enjoy, such as listening to music or being outdoors, to make your workout more enjoyable.

Create a Supportive Environment:
- **Engage family or friends**: Involve your loved ones, encouraging them to join you in Pilates sessions or providing the support you need to stay committed.

- **Designate a workout space**: Set up a designated area at home for

Pilates, creating a space that motivates you to practice regularly.

Prioritize Self-Care:
- **Self-awareness**: Recognize the importance of self-care and view Pilates as a form of self-care that contributes to your overall well-being.

- **Allocate 'me time':** Dedicate time for yourself, incorporating Pilates into this 'me time' as a way to prioritize self-care.

Be Adaptable and Realistic:
- **Flexibility in planning**: Be flexible with your Pilates routine, adjusting it as needed to accommodate unexpected events or changes in your schedule.

- **Realistic expectations**: Set achievable goals and expectations for your Pilates practice, considering your lifestyle and commitments.

Mixing and Matching Exercises

Mixing and matching Pilates exercises allow you to create diverse and engaging workouts tailored to your fitness goals, preferences, and available time. Here's a guide on how to effectively mix and match Pilates exercises:

Understand Exercise Categories:
- **Mat exercises**: Include exercises that require only a mat, focusing on bodyweight resistance and targeted muscle engagement.

- **Reformer exercises**: Incorporate exercises using a Pilates Reformer, utilizing springs for resistance and varied movements.

Consider Muscle Groups:
- **Full-body workout**: Design a routine that engages all major muscle groups, ensuring a comprehensive workout.

- **Isolated muscle focus**: Create workouts that emphasize specific muscle groups, allowing for targeted strengthening and toning.

Choose Exercises Based on Goals:
- **Flexibility and mobility**: Include exercises that focus on stretching and improving range of motion, promoting flexibility and joint mobility.

- **Strength and endurance**: Integrate exercises that challenge muscle strength and endurance, fostering muscular growth and stamina.

Alternate Between Intensity Levels:
- **High-intensity exercises**: Incorporate high-intensity Pilates movements that elevate heart rate and challenge endurance, providing a cardiovascular benefit.

- **Low-intensity exercises**: Include low-impact exercises that focus on form, control, and muscle engagement, allowing for active recovery.

Mix Equipment and Props:

- **Reformer and mat exercises**: Blend exercises using both the Reformer and mat to maximize versatility and target muscle groups from various angles.

- **Incorporate props:** Use props like resistance bands, stability balls, and magic circles to add challenge and variety to your routine.

Create Workout Themes:

- **Core-centric workout:** Design a workout with a primary focus on core-strengthening exercises, enhancing stability and posture.

- **Flexibility flow**: Develop a routine that emphasizes fluid movements and stretches, promoting increased flexibility and relaxation.

Rotate Exercises Regularly:
- **Weekly rotation:** Change your workout routine weekly, incorporating new exercises and variations to keep your workouts fresh and engaging.

- **Monthly progressions**: Plan monthly progressions, gradually increasing intensity and difficulty to ensure continual growth and challenge.

Listen to Your Body:
- **Individualize workouts**: Modify exercises based on your fitness level, any injuries, or physical limitations to ensure a safe and effective workout.

- **Avoid overexertion**: Be mindful of your body's signals and adjust the intensity or duration of exercises to prevent burnout or injury.

MODIFICATIONS AND SAFETY GUIDELINES

Understanding Modifications:

- **Purpose of modifications**: Modifications in Pilates are adjustments to exercises that accommodate individual abilities, injuries, or limitations while maintaining the essence and benefits of the movement.

- **Tailoring to needs**: Modifying exercises helps in personalizing the workout, making it accessible to a broader audience and preventing potential injuries.

Common Modifications:
- **Reducing intensity**: Beginners or individuals with limited mobility can start with fewer repetitions or simpler variations of an exercise to

gradually build strength and flexibility.

- **Using props**: Incorporating props like resistance bands, blocks, or stability balls can aid in providing support, adding resistance, or enhancing range of motion.

- **Adjusting range of motion**: Adapting the range of motion in an exercise allows individuals to work within their comfortable and safe limits, preventing strain or discomfort.

- **Changing body position**: Altering body position can reduce or increase the intensity of an exercise, making it suitable for different fitness levels.

Safety Guidelines:
- **Consult a healthcare professional**: Prior to starting Pilates, especially if you have pre-existing health conditions or

injuries, consult with a healthcare provider for guidance and clearance.

- **Qualified instruction**: Practice under the guidance of a certified Pilates instructor who can provide proper cues, corrections, and modifications to ensure safe and effective workouts.

- **Body awareness**: Listen to your body and avoid pushing beyond your limits. Pay attention to any discomfort, pain, or signs of overexertion during the practice.

- **Proper technique:** Focus on mastering the correct technique of each exercise to prevent injuries and maximize the benefits of the workout.

- **Warm-up and cool down**: Always start with a proper warm-up and end with a cool-down to prepare your body for exercise and aid in recovery.

Progression and Gradual Advancement:

- **Gradual progression**: As you gain strength and flexibility, gradually increase the intensity, duration, or complexity of the exercises to ensure consistent improvement.

- **Mindful advancement**: Pay attention to your body's responses, progress at a pace that suits you, and avoid rushing into challenging exercises too soon.

Breath and Alignment:

- **Focus on breathing:** Coordinate your breath with the movements to enhance oxygen flow, energy, and focus throughout the practice.

- **Maintain proper alignment**: Pay attention to maintaining proper spinal alignment and body positioning during exercises to prevent strain or injury.

Hydration and Nutrition:

- **Stay hydrated**: Drink water before, during, and after your Pilates session to prevent dehydration and muscle cramps.

- **Balanced nutrition**: Ensure a balanced diet rich in proteins, carbohydrates, fats, vitamins, and minerals to support your overall fitness and energy levels.

Tailoring Pilates for Individual Needs

Tailoring Pilates for individual needs ensures that the practice is effective, enjoyable, and aligns with the specific objectives of the practitioner.

Understanding Individual Needs:

- **Assessing fitness levels**: Evaluate the fitness level of the individual, considering their strength, flexibility, cardiovascular health, and overall physical condition.

- **Identifying goals:** Understand the individual's objectives, whether it's improving posture, building core strength, rehabilitating an injury, or enhancing athletic performance.

- **Considering limitations**: Take into account any pre-existing medical conditions, injuries, or physical limitations that might affect the choice of exercises.

Customization Strategies:
- **Exercise selection**: Choose Pilates exercises that align with the individual's goals, ensuring a focused approach to achieving the desired outcomes.

- **Intensity and progression**: Adjust the intensity, duration, repetitions, and difficulty level of exercises to suit the individual's fitness level and prevent overexertion or under-stimulation.

- **Incorporate variety**: Integrate a diverse range of Pilates exercises to keep the practice engaging, challenging, and effective in targeting different muscle groups.

Targeted Focus Areas:
- **Core strengthening**: Emphasize exercises that target the core muscles, as core strength is fundamental to a successful Pilates practice and supports overall stability.

- **Flexibility and mobility**: Incorporate stretching and mobility exercises to improve range of motion, reduce stiffness, and enhance flexibility.

- **Injury rehabilitation**: Design a program that focuses on rehabilitating injuries, providing gentle movements and modifications to aid in the recovery process.

Adapting for Special Populations:
- **Prenatal and postnatal Pilates**: Modify exercises for pregnant and postpartum individuals to ensure safety and address specific physical changes during and after pregnancy.

- **Seniors and older adults:** Tailor exercises for older adults, considering mobility challenges and focusing on gentle movements that enhance balance, flexibility, and muscle strength.

Individualized Attention:
- **One-on-one sessions**: Provide personalized attention through private sessions, allowing the instructor to focus on the individual's needs and adapt the workout accordingly.

- **Regular assessments**: Conduct regular assessments to track progress, identify areas for improvement, and make necessary adjustments to the workout plan.

Effective Communication:
- **Encourage feedback**: Maintain open communication with the individual, encouraging them to share their experiences, concerns, and preferences during the practice.

- **Educate and inform**: Provide information on the benefits of Pilates, the purpose of specific exercises, and the expected outcomes, fostering a deeper understanding of the practice.

Empowerment and Positivity:
- **Motivational support**: Encourage and motivate the individual throughout their Pilates journey, celebrating their achievements and progress.

- **Build confidence**: Foster a positive and supportive environment that boosts the individual's confidence, empowering them to embrace the practice and strive for their goals.

Addressing Common Health Concerns

Here's a comprehensive guide to addressing common health concerns when practicing Pilates:

Back Pain and Spinal Issues:
- **Consult a professional**: Individuals with chronic or severe back pain should consult a healthcare professional before starting Pilates to determine if it's appropriate and safe.

- **Emphasize proper alignment**: Focus on exercises that promote spinal alignment, strengthen the core, and improve posture, which can help alleviate back pain.

Arthritis and Joint Problems:

- **Low-impact exercises**: Choose low-impact Pilates exercises that are gentle on the joints, providing a safe way to enhance flexibility and muscle strength without exacerbating arthritis symptoms.

- **Avoid straining joints**: Encourage smooth and controlled movements to prevent any excessive stress on the joints, particularly for individuals with arthritis.

Osteoporosis and Bone Health:

- **Consult with a specialist**: Seek guidance from a healthcare provider or physical therapist to determine safe exercises that promote bone health without risking fractures.

- **Focus on weight-bearing exercises**: Incorporate weight-bearing and resistance exercises to enhance bone density while ensuring proper alignment and caution.

Respiratory Conditions:

- **Breath awareness**: Emphasize exercises that focus on breath awareness, helping individuals with respiratory conditions improve their lung capacity and respiratory control.

- **Modify intensity**: Adjust the intensity and pace of exercises to accommodate individuals with respiratory conditions, ensuring a comfortable and safe workout.

Postpartum Concerns:

- **Wait for clearance**: Ensure individuals receive medical clearance from their healthcare provider before starting postnatal Pilates to verify that they are ready for physical activity.

- **Target pelvic floor and core:** Incorporate exercises that specifically target pelvic floor muscles and core strength, aiding in postpartum recovery and strengthening.

Cardiovascular Issues:
- **Monitor heart rate:** Encourage individuals with cardiovascular issues to monitor their heart rate during Pilates and maintain a moderate intensity, avoiding overexertion.

- **Incorporate low-impact exercises**: Emphasize low-impact Pilates exercises to provide cardiovascular benefits without placing excessive stress on the heart.

Chronic Health Conditions:
- **Medical guidance:** Advocate for individuals with chronic health conditions to consult their healthcare provider before starting Pilates, ensuring that the practice is safe and suitable for their condition.

- **Regular communication**: Maintain open communication with individuals regarding their health concerns, progress, and any changes in their condition to adapt exercises accordingly.

Injury Prevention:

- **Proper technique**: Stress the importance of proper technique and form to prevent injuries during Pilates exercises.

- **Guidance from professionals**: Encourage individuals to seek guidance from certified Pilates instructors who can provide appropriate modifications and ensure safe execution of exercises.

NUTRITION AND PILATES: A COMPREHENSIVE GUIDE

The Role of Nutrition in Pilates Practice

Pre-Workout Nutrition

Pre-workout nutrition lays the foundation for a successful Pilates session. What you consume before exercising impacts your energy levels, focus, and endurance. Here's a comprehensive look at optimizing your pre-workout nutrition for Pilates:

Timing of Pre-Workout Nutrition:
- **Meal timing**: Consume a balanced meal 2-3 hours before your Pilates session to allow for proper digestion and nutrient absorption.

- **Snacking closer to the session**: If a meal is not possible, have a light snack 30-60 minutes before Pilates to provide a quick energy boost.

Components of Pre-Workout Nutrition:

- **Carbohydrates**: Choose complex carbohydrates like whole grains, fruits, and vegetables for sustained energy throughout your Pilates session.

- **Proteins**: Incorporate lean proteins such as chicken, fish, or plant-based sources like legumes to support muscle function and recovery.

- **Healthy fats**: Include sources of healthy fats like nuts, seeds, and avocados to aid in satiety and sustained energy.

Hydration:

- **Pre-hydrate**: Drink adequate water before your session to ensure you start your Pilates practice in a well-hydrated state.

- **Electrolyte balance**: Consider hydrating with electrolyte-rich beverages to maintain electrolyte balance, especially if you'll be sweating during the session.

Example Pre-Workout Meals and Snacks:

- **Meal option**: Grilled chicken with quinoa and steamed vegetables.

- **Snack option**: Greek yogurt with a small banana and a handful of almonds.

Post-Workout Nutrition

Post-workout nutrition is crucial for recovery and muscle repair after a Pilates session. Here's a comprehensive guide on how to optimize your post-workout nutrition:

Timing of Post-Workout Nutrition:
- **Golden hour:** Consume a balanced meal or snack within 30-60 minutes after your Pilates session to facilitate muscle recovery and replenish energy stores.

Components of Post-Workout Nutrition:
- **Proteins:** Prioritize high-quality protein sources like eggs, lean meats, or plant-based proteins to aid in muscle repair and growth.

- **Carbohydrates:** Include complex carbohydrates to replenish glycogen stores and restore energy levels. Choose starchy vegetables, fruits, or whole grains.

- **Healthy fats:** Incorporate sources of healthy fats like nuts, seeds, or olive oil to support overall health and satiety.

Hydration:
- **Rehydration**: Consume fluids to rehydrate your body after sweating during the session. Water is a simple and effective choice.

Example Post-Workout Meals and Snacks:
- **Meal option**: Grilled salmon with sweet potatoes and a side of steamed broccoli.

- **Snack option**: Protein smoothie with whey protein, spinach, banana, and almond milk.

Maintaining a Balanced Diet

Here's a comprehensive guide to help you achieve and sustain a well-rounded, nutritious diet:

Components of a Balanced Diet:
- **Proteins**: Include lean meats, poultry, fish, eggs, legumes, and plant-based proteins to support muscle growth, repair, and overall body function.

- **Carbohydrates**: Opt for whole grains, fruits, vegetables, and legumes to provide energy and essential nutrients.

- **Fats**: Incorporate healthy fats from sources like nuts, seeds, avocados, and oily fish for heart health and overall well-being.

- **Fiber**: Ensure a sufficient intake of fiber from whole grains, fruits, vegetables, and legumes to support digestion and maintain a healthy weight.

- **Vitamins and minerals**: Consume a variety of colorful fruits and vegetables to obtain a spectrum of vitamins and minerals that are essential for various bodily functions.

- **Water consumption**: To stay hydrated and maintain biological functioning, drink enough water throughout the day.

Portion Control and Moderation:
- **Mindful portions**: Be conscious of portion sizes to avoid overeating and maintain a healthy weight.

- **Moderation**: Enjoy a wide variety of foods in moderation, balancing indulgences with healthier choices.

Meal Planning and Preparation:
- **Weekly planning**: Plan your meals for the week, incorporating a mix of

proteins, carbohydrates, and fats to create balanced and nutritious meals.

- **Batch cooking**: Prepare meals in batches, saving time and ensuring you have healthy options readily available during the week.

Listening to Your Body:
- **Intuitive eating**: Listen to your body's hunger and fullness cues to eat when hungry and stop when satisfied.

- **Restrictions should be avoided**: Restrictive diets and eating habits can result in nutrient deficits and a negative relationship with food.

Consulting a Nutrition Professional:
- **Registered Dietitian**: Consider consulting a registered dietitian for personalized guidance, especially if you have specific health concerns or dietary goals.

Adapting to Lifestyle Changes:
- **Flexibility and adaptation**: Be flexible in your dietary choices to adapt to changing circumstances, travel, social events, and lifestyle adjustments.

STAYING MOTIVATED AND OVERCOMING CHALLENGES

Find Your Why:
- **Define your purpose**: Understand the reasons behind practicing Pilates. It could be for improved flexibility, rehabilitation, stress relief, or general fitness. Understanding your mission will encourage commitment.

Set Short-Term and Long-Term Goals:
- **Break down your goals:** Divide your Pilates objectives into achievable short-term goals and broader long-term aspirations. Celebrate milestones along the way to maintain motivation.

Mix Up Your Routine:
- **Variety is key**: Spice up your Pilates routine by introducing new exercises, props, or workout

locations. A change in routine prevents boredom and keeps you excited about your practice.

Track Your Progress:
- **Document your journey**: Keep a Pilates journal to note your progress, how exercises feel, and any improvements in strength or flexibility. Reflecting on your growth can be highly motivating.

Seek Inspiration:
- **Follow influencers**: Engage with Pilates enthusiasts and professionals on social media. Their progress, tips, and enthusiasm can inspire you to stay on track.

Join a Community:
- **Connect with fellow practitioners**: Join Pilates classes or online communities where you can share your experiences, ask questions, and draw motivation from a supportive group.

Remind Yourself of Benefits:
- **Stay mindful of gains**: Regularly remind yourself of the benefits Pilates offers—better posture, improved core strength, reduced stress, and more. Remembering the positives can reignite your motivation.

Schedule Workouts:
- **Prioritize your practice**: Treat Pilates sessions as essential appointments in your calendar. Make a commitment to yourself and prioritize your well-being.

Visualize Success:
- **Imagine your goals**: Picture yourself achieving your Pilates goals. Visualization can reinforce your determination and drive to reach them.

Seek Professional Guidance:
- **Consult an instructor**: If you're feeling stuck, consider consulting a Pilates instructor for guidance and

motivation. Their expertise can reignite your passion for the practice.

Embrace Setbacks:
- **Learn from challenges**: Accept that setbacks and challenges are a natural part of any journey. Embrace them as learning experiences, allowing them to fuel your determination to overcome.

Setting and Adjusting Your Goals

Setting and adjusting your goals in Pilates is fundamental for progress and satisfaction in your practice. Here's a comprehensive guide to help you set, evaluate, and adapt your Pilates goals effectively:

Understand SMART Goals:
- **Specific**: Clearly define what you want to achieve in Pilates.

- **Measurable**: Establish metrics to track your progress and achievements.

- **Achievable**: Ensure your goals are realistic and attainable within your abilities and resources.

- **Relevant**: Align your goals with your overall Pilates objectives and purpose.

- **Time-bound**: Set a clear timeframe within which you aim to achieve each goal.

Identify Short-Term and Long-Term Goals:
- **Short-term goals**: These could be achieving a specific Pilates pose or improving core strength within a month.

- **Long-term goals**: Consider broader objectives like mastering an advanced Pilates routine or achieving a certain level of flexibility in six months to a year.

Prioritize Your Goals:
- **Primary objectives**: Focus on a few core goals at a time to avoid feeling overwhelmed. Once you achieve them, set new ones.

Evaluate and Adjust Goals Regularly:
- **Progress assessment**: Regularly assess your progress towards your goals. If needed, modify your goals to reflect your current abilities and circumstances.

Celebrate Milestones:
- **Acknowledge achievements**: Celebrate reaching milestones along your journey, whether big or small. It's a way to stay motivated and inspired.

Be Adaptable:
- **Be open to change**: Be willing to adjust your goals as you grow and evolve in your Pilates practice. Your

goals should reflect your current abilities and aspirations.

Consult with a Professional:
- **Instructor's input**: Seek guidance from a Pilates instructor in setting realistic and beneficial goals based on your fitness level and objectives.

Incorporate Variety:
- **Diversify your goals**: Include a mix of goals related to strength, flexibility, balance, and endurance. A well-rounded approach ensures holistic progress.

Track Your Progress:
- **Use a journal**: Record your progress regularly, noting improvements, setbacks, and how you felt during each session. Analyzing this data can guide your goal adjustments.

Stay Committed:
- **Maintain dedication**: Remind yourself of your goals daily and

recommit to them regularly to ensure you stay on track.

Seek Encouragement:
- **Share your goals**: Share your Pilates goals with a friend or your instructor. Their encouragement can motivate you to push towards your targets.

Stay Realistic:
- **Achievable aspirations**: Ensure your goals are challenging but realistic, considering your current fitness level, time commitment, and lifestyle.

Staying Consistent with Your Pilates Practice

Here's a comprehensive guide on how to maintain consistency in your Pilates practice and make it a part of your routine:

Establish a Routine:
- **Set a schedule**: Allocate specific times during the week for your Pilates practice and treat them as non-negotiable appointments.

Start Slow and Build Gradually:
- **Begin with manageable frequency**: Initiate your practice with a realistic number of sessions per week. As you build strength and endurance, gradually increase the frequency.

Mix In Short Sessions:
- **Incorporate brief workouts**: On busy days, opt for shorter Pilates sessions to ensure you're still consistent with your practice.

Integrate Pilates into Your Lifestyle:
- **Incorporate it daily:** Incorporate Pilates principles and exercises into your daily life, whether it's focusing on posture while sitting or doing a quick stretch during breaks.

Create a Dedicated Space:
- **Designate a Pilates area**: Set up a designated space for your practice at home, making it easier to transition into your routine without any setup delays.

Prioritize Self-Care:
- **Recognize its importance:** Understand that Pilates is a form of self-care, promoting both physical and mental well-being. Prioritize it in your schedule accordingly.

Mix Up Your Workouts:
- **Include variety:** Combine different Pilates styles, exercises, or props to keep your routine engaging and prevent monotony.

Accountability and Support:
- **Exercise with a buddy**: Partner with a friend or family member for Pilates sessions, providing mutual accountability and support.

Set Reminders:
- **Use technology**: Set reminders on your phone or fitness apps to prompt you about your scheduled Pilates sessions.

Celebrate Your Progress:
- **Acknowledge   dedication**: Regularly recognize and celebrate your consistency in maintaining your Pilates routine. It's a commendable accomplishment.

Adapt to Your Lifestyle:
- **Flexibility is key**: Be flexible in your approach, adjusting your Pilates schedule to fit changes in your daily routine or lifestyle.

Listen to Your Body:
- **Rest when needed**: If you're feeling fatigued or your body needs rest, honor those signals and give yourself the time to recover.

Overcoming Plateaus and Boredom

Plateaus and boredom are common challenges in any fitness regimen, including Pilates. Here's a comprehensive guide to help you overcome these hurdles and revitalize your Pilates practice:

Identify the Cause of Plateaus:
- **Evaluate your routine:** Assessyour current Pilates regimen, including exercises, intensity, and frequency, to determine if you've reached a plateau.

Adjust Your Routine:
- **Change your exercises**: Introduce new Pilates exercises or modify existing ones to challenge different muscle groups and prevent plateaus.

Increase Intensity:
- **Progress gradually**: Gradually increase the intensity of your Pilates workouts by adding resistance,

increasing repetitions, or extending your session durations.

Incorporate Advanced Techniques:
- **Progress to advanced exercises**: If you've mastered foundational exercises, progress to more advanced Pilates techniques that provide a higher level of difficulty and engagement.

Consult a Professional:
- **Seek expert guidance**: Consider working with a Pilates instructor to design a more challenging routine and provide guidance on overcoming plateaus.

Cross-Train:
- **Mix in other exercises**: Integrate cross-training by incorporating other forms of exercise, such as yoga, cardio, or strength training, to complement your Pilates practice and break through plateaus.

Prioritize Recovery:

- **Allow time for recovery**: Ensure you're giving your body enough time to recover between Pilates sessions, allowing for muscle repair and growth.

Reignite Passion:

- **Rediscover your love for Pilates**: Remind yourself of why you started Pilates in the first place. Sometimes rediscovering your passion can reignite your drive to overcome plateaus.

Combat Boredom with Variety:

- **Change the scenery**: Practice Pilates in different settings—a park, studio, or home—to break the monotony and refresh your mindset.

- **Try new props**: Incorporate various props like stability balls, resistance bands, or Pilates circles to add excitement and a new dimension to your practice.

- **Experiment with classes**: Attend different Pilates classes, each with its unique style and approach, to keep your practice diverse and interesting.

Set Exciting Goals:
- **Create new objectives**: Set challenging yet achievable goals, pushing yourself to progress and break through any performance plateaus.

Practice Mindfulness:
- **Focus on the present**: Practice mindfulness during your Pilates sessions, paying attention to each movement, breath, and sensation. It can elevate your engagement and alleviate boredom.

Take Breaks When Needed:
- **Step back temporarily**: If you're feeling extremely bored or burnt out, take a short break from Pilates. Sometimes, a little hiatus can reignite your enthusiasm.

PILATES FOR SPECIFIC HEALTH CONCERNS

Managing Arthritis and Joint Pain

Arthritis is a condition characterized by inflammation and stiffness in the joints, causing discomfort and limiting mobility. Pilates can be a helpful tool in managing arthritis symptoms and improving joint function.

Here's a comprehensive guide to understanding and utilizing Pilates for managing arthritis and joint pain:

Understanding Arthritis:
- **Different types of arthritis:** Gain knowledge about the various forms of arthritis, including osteoarthritis (OA) and rheumatoid arthritis (RA), to understand their impact on joint health.

Adapting Pilates for Arthritis:
- **Low-impact exercises:** Emphasize low-impact Pilates exercises that are gentle on the joints, such as gentle stretching, controlled movements, and fluid transitions.

- **Focus on joint mobility**: Incorporate exercises that prioritize improving joint mobility and range of motion, promoting flexibility and reducing stiffness.

- **Avoid overexertion**: Ensure exercises are tailored to individual capabilities, avoiding excessive strain on affected joints.

Benefits of Pilates for Arthritis:
- **Strengthening muscles around joints**: Pilates can help strengthen the muscles around affected joints, providing stability and support to reduce pain and improve functionality.

- **Enhanced flexibility**: Pilates exercises enhance flexibility, allowing for improved joint movement and reduced stiffness.

- **Mind-body connection**: Pilates encourages a mind-body connection, fostering relaxation and alleviating stress associated with arthritis.

Consulting a Professional:
- **Certified instructors**: Consider working with a certified Pilates instructor experienced in adapting exercises for individuals with arthritis, ensuring a safe and effective practice.

- **Medical consultation**: Consult a healthcare professional before starting a Pilates routine, especially if arthritis symptoms are severe or if additional medical guidance is needed.

Sample Pilates Exercises for Arthritis:

- **Gentle stretching**: Incorporate gentle stretching exercises such as neck stretches, shoulder rolls, and wrist circles to promote joint mobility.

- **Leg slides**: Perform leg slides to gently work the hips and knees, supporting mobility without excessive strain.

- **Pelvic tilts**: Engage in pelvic tilts to strengthen the core muscles and support the lower back.

Improving Bone Health and Osteoporosis

Osteoporosis is a condition characterized by weakened bones, making them more susceptible to fractures and breaks. Pilates, with its focus on weight-bearing exercises, can aid in improving bone health and managing osteoporosis. Here's a comprehensive guide on utilizing Pilates for this purpose:

Understanding Osteoporosis:
- **Bone structure and health**: Gain a comprehensive understanding of bone structure, bone loss in osteoporosis, and the implications for overall health.

- **Risk factors**: Identify risk factors associated with osteoporosis, including age, gender, family history, and lifestyle choices.

Adapting Pilates for Osteoporosis:
- **Weight-bearing exercises**: Integrate weight-bearing Pilates exercises, where the body supports its weight against gravity, to stimulate bone growth and improve bone density.

- **Spinal alignment and safety**: Emphasize proper spinal alignment and safety during exercises to reduce the risk of fractures.

Benefits of Pilates for Osteoporosis:
- **Strengthens bones and muscles**: Weight-bearing Pilates exercises strengthen bones and muscles, promoting better bone density and reducing the risk of fractures.

- **Enhanced balance and posture**: Pilates focuses on balance and posture, crucial for individuals with osteoporosis to prevent falls and fractures.

Consulting a Professional:
- **Certified instructors**: Work with a certified Pilates instructor knowledgeable in adapting exercises for individuals with osteoporosis to ensure safe and effective workouts.

- **Medical consultation**: Seek guidance from a healthcare professional to assess the severity of osteoporosis and tailor a Pilates routine accordingly.

Sample Pilates Exercises for Osteoporosis:

- **Plank variations**: Incorporate modified plank exercises to engage the core muscles and support bone health without excessive strain.

- **Squats**: Perform squats with proper form to strengthen leg muscles and promote bone density in the lower body.

- **Bridge exercises**: Engage in bridge exercises to target the back, glutes, and hips, supporting bone health in the spine and lower body.

Enhancing Mobility and Flexibility

Mobility and flexibility are vital components of a healthy and active lifestyle, promoting better movement and preventing injuries. Pilates, with its emphasis on fluid and controlled movements, is an excellent way to enhance mobility and flexibility.

Here's a comprehensive guide to understanding and utilizing Pilates for this purpose:

Understanding Mobility and Flexibility:
- **Definition and significance**: Define mobility and flexibility, understanding their importance in daily activities and physical fitness.

- **Factors influencing mobility**: Identify factors such as age, sedentary lifestyle, and medical conditions that can affect mobility and flexibility.

Adapting Pilates for Mobility and Flexibility:

- **Dynamic stretching:** Incorporate dynamic stretching and fluid movements in Pilates routines to improve range of motion and flexibility.

- **Full-body engagement**: Design Pilates exercises that engage multiple muscle groups, promoting better overall mobility and flexibility.

Benefits of Pilates for Mobility and Flexibility:

- **Improved range of motion**: Pilates promotes an improved range of motion in joints and muscles, essential for daily activities and athletic performance.

- **Reduced muscle tension**: Regular Pilates practice helps reduce muscle tension and stiffness, contributing to enhanced flexibility and mobility.

Consulting a Professional:
- **Certified instructors**: Work with a certified Pilates instructor who can design a tailored program focusing on mobility and flexibility, addressing your specific needs and goals.

- **Physical assessment**: Conduct a physical assessment to identify areas of limited mobility and flexibility, guiding the design of a targeted Pilates routine.

Sample Pilates Exercises for Mobility and Flexibility:
- **Spinal rotations**: Perform spinal rotations and twists to improve mobility in the spine, promoting better movement and flexibility.

- **Hip flexor stretches:** Incorporate hip flexor stretches to enhance hip mobility, beneficial for activities like walking and running.

- **Shoulder stretches**: Engage in shoulder stretches to improve upper body mobility and reduce tension in the neck and shoulders.

Alleviating Back Pain

Back pain is a prevalent health concern that can significantly impact daily life and overall well-being. Pilates, known for its benefits in strengthening the core and promoting spinal alignment, can be highly effective in alleviating back pain.

Here's a comprehensive guide on utilizing Pilates for this purpose:

Understanding Back Pain:
- **Types of back pain**: Understand different types of back pain, including lower back pain, upper back pain, and sciatica, to identify

the underlying causes and appropriate approaches to relief.

- **Common causes**: Identify common causes of back pain, such as poor posture, muscle strain, herniated discs, or spinal misalignment.

Adapting Pilates for Back Pain:
- **Core-strengthening exercises**: Emphasize core-strengthening Pilates exercises to provide support to the spine and alleviate strain on the back muscles.

- **Spinal alignment:** Incorporate exercises that focus on proper spinal alignment, encouraging better posture and reducing back pain.

Benefits of Pilates for Back Pain:
- **Strengthened core muscles**: Pilates strengthens core muscles, providing better support to the spine and reducing the risk of back pain.

- **Improved posture:** Regular Pilates practice encourages better posture, relieving stress on the back muscles and promoting a pain-free back.

Consulting a Professional:
- **Certified instructors**: Work with a certified Pilates instructor specializing in back pain relief to create a tailored routine that addresses your specific concerns and needs.

- **Medical consultation**: Seek guidance from a healthcare professional to evaluate the severity of your back pain and ensure Pilates is a safe option for you.

Sample Pilates Exercises for Alleviating Back Pain:
- **Cat-cow stretch**: Perform the cat-cow stretch to gently mobilize the spine and alleviate tension in the back muscles.

- **Child's pose**: Engage in the child's pose to stretch the lower back and promote relaxation.

- **Pelvic curls**: Incorporate pelvic curls to strengthen the lower back muscles and improve spinal alignment.

Addressing Stress and Anxiety

Stress and anxiety are prevalent in today's fast-paced world, affecting both physical and mental well-being. Pilates, with its emphasis on controlled movements, breathing, and mindfulness, can be a powerful tool in managing and reducing stress and anxiety.

Here's a comprehensive guide to understanding and utilizing Pilates for this purpose:

Understanding Stress and Anxiety:

- **Definition and impact**: Define stress and anxiety, understanding their impact on the body and mind, and their link to physical tension and discomfort.

- **Identifying triggers**: Recognize common triggers of stress and anxiety, allowing for proactive management and coping strategies.

Adapting Pilates for Stress and Anxiety:
- **Mindful movement**: Integrate mindful movements in Pilates routines, focusing on breath awareness and body sensations to encourage relaxation and reduce stress.

- **Breathing exercises**: Emphasize breathing exercises in Pilates, incorporating deep breathing and rhythmic patterns to promote relaxation and reduce anxiety.

Benefits of Pilates for Stress and Anxiety:

- **Stress reduction**: Pilates, with its focus on mindful movement and controlled breathing, can significantly reduce stress levels, promoting a sense of calm and well-being.

- **Enhanced relaxation**: Engaging in Pilates induces a state of relaxation, reducing muscle tension and aiding in anxiety reduction.

Consulting a Professional:

- **Certified instructors**: Work with a certified Pilates instructor knowledgeable in using Pilates for stress and anxiety management, creating a customized routine that addresses your specific needs.

- **Mental health consultation**: Consider seeking guidance from a mental health professional to integrate Pilates into a comprehensive stress and anxiety management plan.

Sample Pilates Exercises for Stress and Anxiety:

- **Diaphragmatic breathing:** Practice diaphragmatic breathing during Pilates exercises, focusing on deep inhales and exhales to promote relaxation and reduce anxiety.

- **Child's pose:** Incorporate the child's pose to encourage a sense of grounding and tranquility during your Pilates practice.

- **Progressive muscle relaxation:** Integrate progressive muscle relaxation techniques within Pilates exercises to reduce muscle tension and anxiety.

CONCLUSION

Congratulations on completing this enlightening journey through Pilates tailored specifically for women over 50. This book has been your trusted guide, introducing you to a rejuvenating and empowering world of Pilates designed to embrace your wisdom, strength, and grace.

You've explored exercises and principles that honor your unique life stage and cater to your body's evolving needs. Pilates for women over 50 is a transformative experience, offering more than just physical exercise. It's about nurturing a resilient body, a calm mind, and a youthful spirit.

You've learned how Pilates can improve posture, enhance flexibility, strengthen muscles, and foster mental well-being. It's a practice that celebrates the wisdom and beauty that come with age.

However, your journey does not finish here. In fact, it's just the beginning of a lifelong commitment to your well-being. As you continue with Pilates, set new goals, embrace the challenges, and celebrate your achievements. Pilates empowers you to take control of your health, vitality, and overall happiness.

So, dear Pilates enthusiast over 50, revel in the strength you are building, savor the flexibility you are gaining, and delight in the peace you are nurturing. Let Pilates be your fountain of youth, and enjoy every precious moment of this timeless journey.

You are on the path to a healthier, happier, and more fulfilling life. Let the magic of Pilates unfold and enrich your days!

Continuing Your Pilates Practice

Continuing your Pilates practice is about making it a sustainable part of your lifestyle. Here's how you can integrate Pilates seamlessly into your routine:

- **Home Practice**: Set up a comfortable space at home for your Pilates practice. Invest in a quality mat and any necessary equipment. Utilize online resources like instructional videos and tutorials to guide your solo sessions.

- **Join Classes**: Explore local Pilates studios or fitness centers that offer Pilates classes. Group classes provide a supportive community and expert guidance, enhancing your practice.

- **Virtual Classes**: In the digital age, numerous platforms offer virtual Pilates classes. Whether live-streamed or pre-recorded, these classes allow you to maintain a structured practice from the comfort of your home.

- **Combine with Other Activities**: Integrate Pilates with other physical activities like yoga, jogging, or cycling. Pilates can complement various exercises, improving overall fitness and preventing muscle imbalances.

- **Stay Updated**: Keep yourself informed about new developments in Pilates, advancements in techniques, and any modifications that can enhance your practice. Reading books, following reputable websites, and attending workshops can broaden your Pilates knowledge.

- **Connect with Pilates Communities**: Join Pilates communities or forums where you can exchange experiences, ask questions, and stay inspired by the progress of fellow Pilates enthusiasts.

- **Inspire Others**: Share your Pilates journey and experiences with friends and family. Encourage them to try Pilates and witness its positive impact firsthand.

Printed in Great Britain
by Amazon

43443333R00086